CRUDE
BLACK MOLASSES

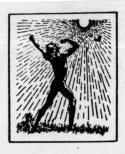

Published and Distributed by
BENEDICT LUST PUBLICATIONS
Box 404 • **New York 10156**

Companion Book to CIDER VINEGAR

AUTHOR'S NOTE

Since drawing attention to the remedial effects of Crude Black Molasses if taken as directed in this booklet, Molasses tablets have appeared on the market. As the liquid, however, plays a certain important part in the treatment, I must point out that molasses in tablet form is unlikely to prove as effective.

Dr. Lust Speaking...

CRUDE
BLACK MOLASSES

The Natural "Wonder-food"

CYRIL SCOTT
and
JOHN LUST,
Naturopath

Benedict Lust Publications

Crude Black Molasses
ISBN 0-87904-010-6
PRINTING HISTORY
Continuously published since the first
Beneficial Book Edition / November 1980
All Rights Reserved
Copyright © 1980 by BENEDICT LUST PUBLICATIONS
Copyright © 1992 by BENEDICT LUST PUBLICATIONS

PUBLISHER'S NOTE: *Where any condition has progressed to a serious stage, or if uncertainty exists as to the seriousness, it is best not to delay timely professional services of a competent physician. This book may not be used in any manner to promote the sale of any products mentioned herein.*

This *Beneficial Book* edition includes every word contained in the original edition of *Crude Black Molasses*. It has been completely reset in a type face designed for easy reading, and was printed from new plates. *Beneficial Books* are published in pocket book form by a division of Benedict Lust Publications, Box 404 Murray Hill, New York, NY 10156 U.S.A.

Printed in the United States of America

Contents

Dr. Lust Speaking...

ABOUT CRUDE BLACK MOLASSES AND YOU

It has been my pleasure to prepare Cyril Scott's classic, *Crude Black Molasses*, for distribution in the U.S.A.

As the author of *Raw Juice Therapy, Drink Your Troubles Away* and *About Raw Juices* the health-building qualities of molasses are especially interesting to me. Molasses is basically a plant juice and thereby takes its place among the fruits, vegetables and herbs that are truly "Nature's Medicines".

Sugar cane, is a deep-rooting grass which burrows as deeply as fifteen feet. It collects trace elements from the soil and gravelly sub-soil. Minerals your system needs.

Without intruding on Mr. Scott's presentation, I'd like to add a bit to this little book about

THAT WONDERFUL BODY OF YOURS

and why these liquid nutrients from plants are your purest and most assimilable forms of nourishment.

If you weigh 145 pounds, no less than 100 pounds represents liquid. It's best you get that liquid as pure as humanly possible. Following is a brief description of some of the roles played by liquid in your body.

Your salivary glands contain juices which digest carbohydrates—beginning in your mouth. They secrete about 3½ pounds in 24 hours. Don't waste your saliva chewing gum, but mix it thoroughly with your food by mastication.

Several glands are in your stomach. Some secrete hydrochloric acid, others pepsin and still others, rennin (to curdle milk). From 8 to 14 pounds of these digestive juices are secreted in 24 hours. Gastric juices convert protein into a digestible form.

The duration of digestion averages from 3 to 5 hours—rice, one hour—pork, 5 hours.

Other digestive juices are produced by glands in the walls of your small intestines. Your alimentary canal is the source of your body's nourishment. Then there are more glands, your pancreas which furnishes important insulin, the antidiabetic hormone, about a pound each day and your liver, the largest of your internal organs. It is a clearing house for some metabolic wastes from your emulsified foods not fit to enter your arterial blood stream. The liver produces a liquid—bile, from 2 to 4 pounds every 24 hours. This is gradually discharged—increasing during digestion—into your duodenum, the connection between your stomach exit and the beginning of your small intestine. Bile is the most alkaline juice in your body. It also has a laxative effect. It assists in the emulsification of fats and stimulates the peristaltic action of the bowels, prevents putrefactive changes in the food and promotes the absorption of fat. When an obstruction forms in the gall duct which carries bile, it deposits in the body's tissues and Jaundice is the result.

Then there is your blood—average amount from 16 to 18 pounds. This is pumped through your vascular system at a rate of about 16 inches per second. Your blood makes its circuit every 30 seconds, or 120 times per hour.

Your two kidneys, situated in the small of your back, perform wonderful work. Urea, representing certain muscular wastes and end products of high protein foods, is formed in the tissues and carried largely to the kidneys where it is separated from the blood and passes into the bladder. The higher your blood pressure, the greater quantity of urine excreted. In Diabetes the quantity is still further increased.

The bladder holds from one to two pints. The normal quantity of urine voided in 24 hours is 40 to 50 ounces. Salt and high protein foods irritate your kidneys and bladder.

Your body truly is a wonderful structure. Take good care of it. Avoid those things you know irritate or damage it if you desire a long life, happy and free from pain. Your normal body temperature is 98.6 F. If for any cause your temperature raises above that, go on a liquid juice fast until it returns to normal.

The mineral content of your food and drink has everything to do with your health. All fertile soil contains the same minerals that make up our bodies. Vegetation extracts those minerals directly from the soil. Our bodies cannot. Vegetation changes those minerals into an organic form, and in that form we can assimilate them.

These minerals are the most important part of our diet. Without them, the proteins, carbohydrates and fats—which are also necessary—cannot provide adequate nutrition. The different digestive juices, hormones and enzymes consist mainly of those minerals in solution.

We must eat foods and drink liquids as close to the form provided by Nature as possible. In Nature's scheme of things there are pure liquids locked in the cells of plants. These have definite therapeutic value. Not only that, they are delightful to eat and drink.

Now, enjoy an important addition to your diet, Blackstrap Molasses. Scott's experiences are convincing facts about the benefits we can expect.

Peace be with you,

John Lust, Editor
New York, NY 10156
November, 1980

ANALYSIS OF MOLASSES

The report on a sample of Molasses used in this country for making silage reveals:

		%
Sucrose	... ...	39.5
Invert sugar	... ...	11.5
Ash	... ...	9.0
Water	... ...	22.5
Organic matter	... ...	17.5

The quantity of insoluble matter is negligible. The 9 percent. ash represents soluble mineral matter largely consisting of potassium and calcium salts.

The United States Department of Agriculture, in Handbook No. 8, COMPOSITION OF FOODS, lists the following content of minerals and vitamins to be found in 100 grams of Crude Blackstrap Molasses:

Calcium	684 mg.
Phosphorus	84 mg.
Iron	16.1 mg.
Sodium	96 mg.
Potassium	2,927 mg.
Magnesium	258 mg.
Thiamine	.11 mg.
Riboflavin	.19 mg.
Niacin	2 mg.

A more detailed analysis of (American Blackstrap Molasses) reveals trace amounts of copper and zinc; furthermore, that the aliment is a rich source of most of the vitamins of the B family with the exception of Vitamin B1. According to the notable diet expert, Gaylord Hauser, it is extremely high in Vitamin B6, in pantothenic acid* and Inositol; and it should be put on one's table as regularly as salt, and used as a sugar substitute on cereals, stirred into milk and eaten instead of jam or jelly.

A most important constituent of Molasses is phosphoric acid: a combined deficiency of this and potassium in the human body "causes a general breakdown of the cells, especially those of the brain and nerves."

Crude Sugar Cane Molasses contains about 50 percent. fruit sugars.

*Pantothenic acid is part of the Vitamin B2 complex. When absent from a chick's diet, the bird develops dermatitis, and degeneration of nerve fibres in the spinal cord also occurs. When rats are fed on a diet lacking in pantothenic acid, necrosis of the suprarenal glands becomes noticeable. (See Appendix II.)

INTRODUCTION

(TO THE FIRST EDITION)

It hardly seems necessary for me to apologize for my frequent allusions in the following pages (1) to the late Dr. Forbes Ross, who, I think, was the first English doctor to draw attention to the prophylactic and curative properties in Crude Black Molasses, (2) to Mr. James Persson of Palmerston N., New Zealand, who, having been cured of a serious disease by this valuable substance, altruistically resolved to supply it at a very low price for the benefit of his fellows. To Mr. Persson I am indebted for the brief case-histories published in this booklet. Many of these cures are those imparted to him by the estwhile sufferers direct, others are cases reported to him (and passed on to me) by the increasing number of persons who have resorted to Molasses-therapy with the most gratifying results, among them doctors and clergymen. Although the names of these doctors are known to me, it would not be wise to mention them, for that might be regarded as indirect advertising. Where the Medical Profession is concerned one is constantly treading on dangerous ground, and the desire to be useful is often frustrated by the demands of etiquette, or other considerations somewhat difficult for the layman to understand. For instance, in one of my books I mentioned certain useful preparations by name, only to be accused of subtle advertising. In my more recent book, "Medicine: Rational and Irrational," I therefore avoided this by saying that certain effective remedies for one or two disorders I dealt with were on the market, but I refrained from stating the names. In consequence I was merely taken to task for not being sufficiently explicit; how was a would-be purchaser sure of getting the right remedy if he did not know its name, and the name of the manufacturer? In short, whatever one does is wrong. Again, there are a number of laws and rulings which make it practically impossible for a writer on medical matters to state what he may believe to be the whole truth. If a doctor writes that a particular preparation is definitely harmful, he runs the risk of a libel action. On the other hand if a doctor has found some preparation or invented a formula which has proved effective in curing, say, cancer, he is not permitted to circularize his confréres, for that is denounced as "unprofessional conduct." Nevertheless he is allowed to give the particulars of his treatment to a medical journal—but there is no certainty that they will be published. All this is fully known to doctors themselves yet not to laymen, for whom these

16

pages are largely written. As for a doctor stating that a remedy for a number of chronic and intractable diseases can be procured at any grocers, he would to say the least be likely to become unpopular among the less altruistic of his colleagues. This is a further good reason why in this connection the names of living orthodox physicians cannot be mentioned. But apart from these restrictions and one or two others it is advisable to impose on myself, I as a musical composer with no personal axe to grind can write more or less what I have good reasons for believing to be true. I say advisedly "more or less" because of fairly recent legislation regarding such diseases as cancer, tuberculosis, etc., which may or may not have some bearing on the matter, for to the non-legal mind they are not very clear. To be explicit: no person other than a qualified doctor is allowed to make known that he can cure cancer, tuberculosis and certain diseases specified, nor is any person or firm allowed to advertise a cure for these disorders. (Not that such rulings can apply to myself as I am neither a practitioner nor an advertiser of any sort.) But here we are faced with a curious situation: the Cancer Research Ring affirm that so far no cure for cancer has yet been discovered. Yet what is precisely meant by a cure; a formula that will *exclusively* cure cancer in practically all patients, or a "something" that will cure a variety of diseases including cancer, or again a substance that so promotes health that, where a cancer is exhibited, it automatically vanishes? As the Cancer Research Ring and the Orthodox Medical Profession have never clearly provided the answers to these questions, speculation on the subject becomes useless. But this must be said; in view of the dictum that no cure for cancer has been discovered, the Profession is obliged to fall back on the assumption that all cases said to be cured by whatever means (excluding surgery and radium) could never have been genuine cancer but merely growths wrongly diagnosed. As to how far the Law does or can be stretched to uphold this dictum I am unable to gauge. But in any event, if I mention cases *said* to be cancer or tuberculosis, it is with reservation—for which I here apologize to the doctors concerned—that faulty diagnosis may have led to their being thus defined; Mr. Persson himself never stated otherwise.

THE AUTHOR.

CRUDE BLACK MOLASSES

1
MOLASSES NOT A PATENT FOOD

We live in an age of "wonder-drugs" and patent foods, not to mention the large variety of patent medicines, all of which are very lucrative propositions. Many of the patent foods, mostly sold at health-food stores, are· useful to counteract the baneful effects of a diet deficient in vitamins and mineral salts. As for the "wonder-drugs" they have their day and then fall out of repute because, being advertised with a flourish of trumpets, they come to be used indiscriminately, and

19

hence, in many cases, do more harm than good.* Even the use of patent food can be overdone on the assumption that one cannot have too much of a good thing! Yet although I have called Molasses a "wonder-food" by way of emphasis there is nothing whatever patent about it, and in most countries not suffering from post-war food shortage, it can be obtained at any grocery at a negligible cost. The unfortunate fact that it is not procurable in this country (Great Britain) except by farmers for the purpose of making silage, does not mean that it will never be procurable when times have become more normal and when the public, the naturopaths and the less orthodox physicians have been made fully aware of its curative and prophylactic properties. As a step to this desideratum I recently wrote a short series of articles in that widely read journal, "Health for All," and, judging from the avalanche of letters I received, it seemed desirable and expedient to enlarge on the subject in the form of the present booklet.

Already, before the first Great War, the late Dr. Forbes Ross drew attention to the value of Molasses in connection with cancer.* He pointed out that workers on sugar-cane, plantations who were constantly sucking the crude sugar, seldom if ever were known to suffer from that dread disease. He attributed this to the large

* Dr. Leon Goldman, Forman Friend and Lester M. Mason, of the University of Cincinnati College of Medicine, examined 350 patients and found 16 reacted unfavourably to contact with penicillin, men more than women.

Their article in the journal of the American Medical Association advised, "use penicillin only where and when indicated ... not indiscriminately for everything."

* See Appendix.

precentage of potassium salts in unrefined sugar-cane; his contention being that the cause of cancer was a deficiency of potash in the human cells and blood. I have dealt with his contentions in some detail in my earlier books and cannot repeat myself in these pages. Suffice it to say that although Dr. Forbes Ross's numerous cures of cancer, together with the book he wrote on the subject, did not receive at the time the recognition they deserved, several eminent physicians of various schools have since come to uphold his views.

I will now without further preamble, proceed to deal with the comparatively large number of diseases which have yielded to Molasses-therapy.

2
GROWTHS

As already implied, my attention was more fully drawn to the curative and prophylactic elements in Crude Black Molasses by one of my numerous correspondents, Mr. James Persson, of Palmerston N., New Zealand. The circumstances are as follows: Some years ago Mr. Persson was broken in health and unable to do even the lightest work. He was suffering from a growth in the bowels, hardened valves of the heart, blocked bronchial tubes, constipation, indigestion, pyorrhoea, sinus trouble and weak nerves. In addition to this array of symptoms, he was losing weight, and his hair had turned white. Despite consulting doctors and specialists his condition was getting steadily worse. Then one day he heard of a Mr. S. who happened to be a neighbour of the postman, from whom he got the details I will now mention. Mr. S. has suffered from an inoperable growth in the bowels; in other words, he had been opened up by the surgeons, and then stitched up again, his condition being regarded as so hopeless that even the idea of surgical interference was abandoned. Thus, he was discharged from hospital, and only given seven weeks to live. However, he was subsequently induced by an acquaintance to try the effect of taking Molasses; with the astonishing result that far from dying within the seven weeks, he finally made a complete recovery. On hearing of this remarkable case, Mr. Persson decided to try the treatment himself—and not only did the growth in his bowels disappear, together with all his other troubles (and this after seven years' suffering), but his hair, which was white when he started the treatment, actually regained its original colour and assumed a more healthy appearance in every respect. It should be mentioned that Mr. Persson is over sixty.

Having proved for himself the curative value of Molasses, he resolved to supply the aliment at 4½d. per lb. so as to keep down the price, seeing that chemists were selling a *medicated* variety at a much higher figure, and thereby spoiling the substance while pretending to improve it. But I shall have something more to say about this later on. Meanwhile, I should repeat here that Mr. Persson's activities were instrumental in bringing him into contact, either directly or indirectly, with a very large number of sufferers from various diseases, including growths. For Mr. S's cure, and Mr. Persson's own cure having become known, the demand for Molasses was such that Mr. Persson was at one time supplying a ton of it a month, and is now supplying even more.

As growths are serious conditions for which the orthodox medico can only suggest radium or the knife, I am dealing with these in my first section.

Among the numerous cases cured solely by Molasses-therapy are growths of the uterus, growths of the breast, further instances of intestinal growth, also numerous cases of growths of the tongue, diagnosed as malignant. One man with a fibroid growth of the tongue was in such a condition that he was unable to speak. But by dint of repeatedly holding Molasses in his mouth and also taking it internally (see Section 24), the growth came away and the man was cured. And yet this merely bears out the late Dr. Forbes Ross's contention that growths of the tongue (he used the word cancer) had been cured by sucking this natural aliment. As for tumours, fibroid growths in various sites of the body, these, according to Mr. Persson and to reports received by him, have withered away without any other measures than that of taking Molasses internally and using it in the form of poultices.

A recent case of uterine growth may now be mentioned in some detail. The sufferer visited Mr. Persson in a very distressed frame of mind. She had been told by the doctors that she was suffering from cancer, and could not be expected to live for more than about six weeks. The diagnosis may have been incorrect, but in any case her doctors took a very serious view of her condition, for she had lost much weight and suffered

25

from severe haemorrhages. Having heard of Molasses for growths, she consequently applied to Mr. Persson for a quantity, which she proceeded to take via the mouth, and also to use in blood-warm water as a douche. (See pp. 13,29,30). Some months after she had started the treatment she called to see Mr. Persson again; and he reports that she was so changed for the better in every way that he could hardly believe it was the same woman. The bleeding had ceased, she had regained her normal weight, her colour was healthy, and she confessed to feeling "wonderful."

Here is another case worthy to mention. Mrs. M—. Breast growth. Given two months to live. After employing Molasses-therapy, the growth disappeared, and she was perfectly well. Many months elapsed. No recurrence.

Mr. Persson writes: "Many sufferers, after taking Molasses for some time, cough up rotten growths." He then, among others, gives the case of a man said to be suffering from cancer of the gullet. Breath very foul until lately. This unfortunate man had to be fed by means of a tube. He is treating himself with Molasses. Has already coughed up "a rotten lump about the size of a small egg, and his breath does not smell bad any more." My correspondent adds: "I have come across some terrible cases, yet wonderful to relate, they have been cured by Molasses."

3
STROKES

According to "The Biochemic System of Medicine," the majority of diseases that are curable at all, are simply due to a deficiency of certain of the mineral salts. It is therefore no surprise to students of this System that paralytic strokes have yielded to Molasses-therapy, seeing that the aliment is so especially rich in a variety of these mineral salts. Where paralysis is exhibited, unless due to accident, there is a lack of calcium, potassium and magnesium in the body; and all these salts are present in assimilable form in Crude Black Molasses.

Now the general supposition is that when a person has had two strokes, the third one will kill him or her, as the case may be. And yet it need not be so, or at any rate not invariably, as the following brief case-history reveals: Mr. X, an elderly man, had had two strokes and was completely paralysed down one side of his body. He then tried Molasses-therapy—with the gratifying result that he *recovered the use of all his limbs*, and became completely fit, much to the astonishment of his doctor and his friends. Nor is this by any means an isolated case, and if I have selected it out of many others, it is because it happens to be a particularly bad one.

The question of paralytic strokes gives one much food for reflection, and I think it is not going too far to say that if people would make Molasses a part of their daily diet there would be fewer cases of this dreadful affliction.

4
ARTHRITIS

Dr. Forbes Ross maintained that there was a certain connection between arthritis and cancer, the reason being that both cancer and arthritis arose from the same cause viz., a deficiency of potassium salts in the human organism. Whether he was entirely correct is open to opinion, for cancer is apt to develop where the sufferer lives in a house situated over an underground stream, or at a point where two underground watercourses cross. But even so, one may still ask whether malignancy would eventuate if the victim were not suffering from a deficiency of potassium salts? In any case, Dr. Forbes Ross would seem to have proved his point in so far that he cured cases of arthritis with precisely the same measures that he cured cancer and that was with potassium salts prepared in an assimilable form. Bearing this in mind it is not difficult to see why a substance (Molasses) which is especially rich in potassium, should not be effective in curing arthritis as well as bodily growths. Moreover, the proof is to hand. Many sufferers who could only hobble about with the aid of sticks, were able to throw the latter away after they had taken a course of Molasses in the prescribed manner.* To facilitate and accelerate the cure, a little *flowers of sulphur* mixed with black treacle were taken every night—in short, the old "brimstone and treacle mixture," immortalized by Dickens in "Nicholas Nickleby."!

In cases where the joints were badly swollen, excellent results have been obtained by bathing them with Molasses mixed with creosote—though Mr. Persson himself did not advocate this procedure as an adjunct to the internal treatment, the idea having apparently originated with certain doctors.

Since the first edition of this booklet was published, such remarkable reports have come in from people in this country (Great Britain) who have been able to employ the treatment with Molasses alone, that it is not extravagant to say that Molasses is THE cure *par excellence* for arthritis. Here are some of the cases, spectacular in the rapidity of the cures.

Lady, turned 70. Complete fixation of hip joints for three years. Knees could not be flexed. Much pain and

* See Section 24, p. 81.

fatigue. Injections given by allopathic doctor, but with no beneficial results whatever. Finally a specialist suggested a costly operation, but could not promise a success. The patient delcined the operation, heard of the Molasses treatment and decided to try it. After thirty-six doses, she could walk without sticks and her knees had become so flexible that she could even kick her posterior with her heels! Another case, Lady of 40 years of age. Bad arthritis in knees and hip joints. Much pain, unable to walk without sticks. Was induced to try Molasses. After one week was able to swing her legs without pain and to flex her knees. Still another case, though improvement less rapid. Old man. Could only hobble about with the aid of two sticks. Took Molasses in the prescribed manner, and in four weeks was able to discard his sticks. Many more cases could be added did space permit.

It is worthy of note that worry is conducive to arthritis. In fact there are cases where a great shock or worry has caused a temporary relapse. In such cases it is of great importance to continue the treatment, seeing that worry uses up the potassium salts in the blood and tissues, therefore trouble is likely to ensue if these are not replenished. Sugar-cane Molasses is here especially important, as the type made from beet sugar is less rich in phosphates, though it has not been devoid of good results where arthritis is not aggravated by worry. In any case, patients who have taken even the beet variety have noticed a marked improvement in their general health in a surprisingly short time, as also an improvement of the arthritic condition. All the same, it should be stressed that the cane Molasses is much superior to the beet Molasses, and hence should be used if procurable.

5
ULCERS

People whose blood is in perfect condition do not suffer from ulcers, especially from a chronic state of ulceration. It is true that doctors can usually cure isolated abscesses, on the other hand such afflictions as ulcerated legs have proved very difficult to heal by orthodox medical methods; though I do happen to know of one doctor who has cured hundreds of very bad cases with his own particular methods. But that is by the way; we are here concerned with ulcers and ulceration cured by no other means than by Molasses. A few years ago a certain doctor in New Zealand was so much afflicted with ulcers that his own skill proved insufficient to cure them. In fact, this doctor was very ill and would doubtless have remained so had he not heard of the Molasses-treatment and was open-minded enough to try it. The upshot was that after taking Molasses for a given period, all his ulcers vanished and he was restored to excellent health.

According to practitioners of the *Biochemic System of Medicine*, ulcers do not occur unless there is some deficiency of certain mineral salts in the blood and tissues. As Molasses, if taken over the requisite time, makes good that deficiency, it is not surprising to hear that *gastric* ulcers have also yielded to the treatment. Indeed the site of the ulcer is not of great importance, seeing that when the blood and tissues are supplied with the essential salts and vitamins to maintain their health, in many cases the local manifestation of the trouble automatically disappears. As all sensible healers know without the telling it is foolish and futile *merely* to treat the local condition—which is only an effect—without removing the prime cause; the untenable supposition being that the body is not a unity and that the parts can be divided from the whole. The rational method of treatment is, where indicated, to treat both locally and internally, as in the case of external ulcers, and also skin diseases, as the following case shows.

6
DERMATITIS. ECZEMA. PSORIASIS

Mr. L.—Hands very red and swollen with dermatitis. He was induced to soak his hands frequently in water to which some Molasses had been added, and to take Molasses several times a day. The cure was complete in six weeks. This is very different from the suppressive treatment which unfortunately many unenlightened skin specialists advocate; their usual procedure being to use ointments which, although they may cure the local condition are apt later on to give rise to something worse—not uncommonly asthma, as many homoepaths are aware. Seeing that a skin disease is an attempt on the part of Nature to rid the body of certain poisons, to suppress that attempt by smearing on ointments is surely to drive those poisons back into the body and so frustrate Nature. It would not even be wise merely to apply diluted Molasses, despite its healing properties, for it is essential that the patient should take the substance internally at the same time so as to get rid of that condition of the blood and tissues which is primarily responsible for the disorder. Experience over a period of nine years has proved that the Molasses-treatment is a rational and natural-scientific method of curing skin diseases. These include dry eczema, weeping eczema, and even some types of psoriasis.

7
HIGH BLOOD PRESSURE.
ANGINA PECTORIS.
WEAK HEART

High Blood Pressure, according to biochemists of the Dr. Schüssler School, is frequently associated with arteriosclerosis, and like most afflictions that are curable at all, is due to a deficiency of certain of the essential mineral salts. But whether the reader is prepared to accept this dictum or not, the fact remains that the most gratifying results have been obtained in many cases by the Molasses-treatment plus the juice of one lemon a day. How is this to be accounted for without making too much demand on the reader's credulity? Simply by realizing that the cause of high blood pressure lies in the fact that the arteries have lost their elasticity and have got hardened and "blocked," as it were, so that it is difficult for the blood to circulate through them without a much increased effort on the part of the heart. Yet, as we learn from the *Schüssler Biochemic System*, they would not lose their elasticity if one or more of the required mineral salts were not lacking to preserve it. These salts being present in Molasses, that is why cases of high blood pressure have been cured by that aliment. Incidentally, though of great importance, Molasses contains ingredients which are very strengthening to the heart muscles. Also, it would seem, that it contains anti-spasm ingredients, notably magnesium, seeing that Mr. Persson reports cases of angina pectoris being cured by the treatment. As for weak heart, it has been known for a long time by orthodox doctors (though they often forget it) that brown sugar is good for that condition. But Crude Black Molasses is far superior to ordinary sugar for the purpose because of the concentration of mineral salts which it contains.

Mr. Persson reports the cases of a number of men who were not granted licences to drive their cars owing to "bad hearts." After taking Molasses for six weeks they were cured, and able to obtain their licences. Even "hopeless" cases have recovered, as, for instance, the following: The sufferer, a Mr. K., was in such a condition that his doctor said he might live at the most a week. In fact the physicians had intimated that "nothing more could be done for him." Nevertheless after taking Molasses for a time he made a complete recovery—a matter which was considered "an absolute miracle"!

Since writing the above, reports of several gratifying cases in England have come to hand, from which the

38

following may be selected. Lady, aged 63. For some three to four years had suffered from various ailments, and particularly from recurrent heart attacks. The patient would wake in the night with violent palpitation, pain, a feeling of suffocation and fright. The face was hot and flushed. Her doctor prescribed remedies, which gave temporary relief but failed to effect a cure. The patient was growing more and more depressed and dissatisfied with life. She was then sent a copy of the first edition of this book, and contrived to obtain some Molasses. After taking it for several weeks, I received a grateful letter from her saying that she "felt an entirely different woman." No more malaise, no more heart attacks. A further letter from her after several months had passed reported that there had been no return of the trouble. She continued to take the Molasses and was so pleased with the results that she was recommending the treatment to all her ailing friends. Similar cases could be cited did space permit.

I will conclude this section with a brief mention of a case of cardiac thrombosis (blood clot). The sufferer was a railway worker who had been obliged to give up his job for life owing to his condition. He was induced to try the Molasses and was so pleased with the results that he was able to go back to work—a fit man. The potassium and other mineral salts in the aliment had dispersed the clot. I may add that potassium is one of the chief salts used by biochemic practitioners for the cure of thrombosis.

8
CONSTIPATION.
COLITIS

Constipation is the bugbear of civilization, and a goldmine to the manufacturing chemists. The obvious reason is that the bulk of people live on deficiency foods, or what the Americans call processed foods; moreover the advent of the motor-car has caused people to take less exercise. Consequently the chemists advertise hundreds of different kinds of laxatives, and the health-food manufacturers sell quantities and varieties of cereals (in packets) calculated to move the bowels. These are well enough in their way, and useful to counteract the bad effects of deficiency flour; but if it were made compulsory—which God forbid—for people to eat whole-meal bread complete with the wheat germ, these "packet-foods" would be superfluous; nor would I need to draw attention to Molasses as a mild and natural evacuent, which undoubtedly it is.

We are told nowadays that constipation comes from an insufficient amount of bulk and roughage, which dictum is only a half-truth, for a great deal of costive-ness comes from the fact that the bowels have lost tone because they have not been supplied with the necessary mineral salts to cause them to function properly. And here is where Molasses proves so valuable, for the salts it contains help to re-establish muscular tone if taken sufficiently to effect this desideratum. This does not mean that Molasses will cure every case of constipa-tion, especially if sufferers live and have lived for years on a "rubbishy" diet of white bread, meat and boiled vegetables of which all the valuable salts have been thrown down the sink. In such cases other measures are required—not purgatives which make matters worse the longer they are resorted to, but measures which are natural as opposed to medicinal, i.e., assist Nature in a mechanical manner without producing of-fensive manifestations. To be explicit: all that is needed is a teaspoonful of linseed, or even a little more if nec-essary. These seeds should be washed through a sieve or tea-strainer, then swallowed with a little water. Their action is twofold; they swell and produce bulk, and at the same time the oil is liberated and acts as a natural and harmless lubricant. As linseed is no more a poison to human beings than canary seed is a poison to canaries, it can be taken every night without the least harm. In any event, where indicated, it should be taken for at least a month, in that its good effects are cumulative.

I mention this harmless evacuent because if people who are treating themselves with Molasses, say, for heart trouble, imagine they can at the same time wisely take their daily dose of liquid paraffin—that being the fashion at present—they are mistaken, the reason being, so it is now contended, that medicinal paraffin is apt to interfere with the absorption of certain vitamins, and some doctors even go so far as to say it interferes with the absorption of one's food in general.

The value of black treacle as a mild aperient has been recognised by homoeopaths for a long time. The *modus operandi* is to dissolve a teaspoonful of it in a tumbler of water, then sip it while dressing in the morning. Nevertheless Crude Black Molasses is far superior to black treacle for the purpose of producing an evacuation. In obstinate cases a dessertspoonful, or even a tablespoonful, should be taken in warm water, on rising, in addition to the daily doses with meals. The practice should be kept up for four to six weeks to effect the cure.

Colitis is another disease of so-called civilization; though admittedly the name is used to cover a variety of conditions—such as diarrhoea of old people. Reports are to hand of cases cured by taking Molasses internally and using enemas in the following way:

Melt a teaspoonful of Molasses in hot water, then add 3 pts. of water so that the temperature of the enema be blood-heat. To obtain the best effects, enemata may

43

be taken every day for the first week, every other day the second week, and every two days the third week. Then discontinued; *except in cases of bowel-growths*, where persistence may be necessary.

9
VARICOSE VEINS

I was recently told by that remarkable scientist and haematologist, Mme. M. de Chrapowicki, that certain naturopaths in America had been using Molasses for varicose veins, having long since known of its healing properties. The treatment is perfectly rational, seeing that when taken internally it makes good that deficiency of mineral salts which is the prime cause of this annoying and often debilitating condition. Reports of several cures in this country have recently come to hand.

10
SOME MISCELLANEOUS CASES

(1) A boy who had been very dull and backward mentally, was put on to the Molasses-treatment by his father. He is now as bright and healthy as the rest of the family.

(2) An X-ray photograph revealed that a certain man had a patch on his lung. He was induced to try Molasses, and after taking it for a given period was X-rayed a second time; the radiograph showed a complete disappearance of the patch.

(3) A Maori girl was said by the doctors to be suffering from tuberculosis of the lung. But whether the diagnosis was correct, or not, she was undoubtedly in very poor health. After taking a course of Molasses,

her health was restored to normality.

(4) A man was in much pain with a *poisoned finger*. He also had a lump under his arm. The poisoned finger was treated locally with Molasses compresses, and healed in three days. The lump under his arm vanished as the result of taking Molasses internally.

(5) Cases of *sinus trouble* have yielded to the treatment in a most gratifying manner. For this complaint, the substance must be taken internally, and a mild solution of it (proportions the same as for an enema) used as a nasal douche. The same measures have also been found very beneficial in cases of nasal catarrh. Antrum trouble should also be mentioned in this connection.

(6) Mr. Persson reports a case of *erysipelas* cured with Molasses; and the doctor in attendance advised the patient to continue taking the aliment in view of its beneficial result.

(7) Before Mr. Persson took Molasses, he was suffering from pyorrhoea, as already stated. Pyorrhoea is a constitutional disease with local manifestation. The doctors advocate extraction of the teeth so as to liberate the poisons, but the real cause of the trouble lies in a deficiency of certain of the mineral salts, hence Molasses-therapy is more rational and less expensive, and should be tried before drastic measures are adopted. Molasses diluted should be used as a mouthwash as well as taken internally in the prescribed manner. As an adjunct to the treatment the biochemic cell-salts, Kali mur., Calc. flour, Nat. phos., all in the 6^x potency can be taken in a combination tablet (three tablets twice daily). When improving, then Calc. sulph. 6^x and Silica 12^x can be taken concurrently (E. F. W. Powell, D. Sc.).

11
ANAEMIA.
PERNICIOUS ANAEMIA

Considering the amount of assimilable iron and calcium in Molasses, it is not surprising to hear that many cases of anaemia, have been cured by taking the aliment. The orthodox treatment of anaemia, which consists largely in the administration of some preparation of iron in large doses for a long time, is not only unsatisfactory but is often attended with unpleasant results in the form of digestive disturbances. The reason is obvious to all naturopaths, for iron and calcium should be absorbed from some natural food and not from some medicinal preparation however scientific it is supposed to be. As for that grevious form of anaemia known as *pernicious* anaemia, I was not at all astonished to hear that it also had yielded to Molasses therapy and that Mr. Persson was able to report quite a number of cures. Indeed, I hardly expected otherwise, considering some years ago I heard from a lady correspondent that she had been entirely cured of pernicious anaemia by taking, on the advice of a "quack," a dessertspoonful of Fowler's Black Treacle twice daily. As, however, Crude Black Molasses contains a greater concentration of mineral salts than black treacle, theoretically I argued that it should prove even more effective. Thereafter came the reports showing that the theory had proved correct.

12
BLADDER TROUBLES. DIFFICULT URINATION

And apropos of theories: as Molasses has been shown to diminish growths, cause them to drop off, or make them automatically disappear, there is good reason to suppose that the potassium salts in Molasses should prevent or cure prostatic enlargement in elderly men. But although there are cases to hand of bladder trouble and difficult urination, as Mr. Persson is not a doctor and doesn't profess to be one, the exact nature of these cases has not been specified. Nevertheless, some of them do suggest prostate troubles, as, for instance, the following: Old man. Great difficulty in urinating. Was about to enter hospital because of stoppage. Was then urged to take Molasses, and also to chew plenty of parsley. Result—he finally got well and did not have to go into hospital. Other cases of bladder trouble (though they may not have been connected with the prostate) have yielded to Molasses-therapy combined with the imbibing of plenty of parsley juice or parsley water.

13
GALL-STONES

There is a treatment for gall-stones, which consists in taking Molasses in the prescribed manner plus 3-4 teaspoonsful of olive oil every day. This treatment is not so farfetched as may appear on the surface, considering that copper and several of the other minerals to be found in Molasses are used by biochemists of the Schüssler School as remedies for this agonizing condition. As to the olive oil its function is obvious. But were I personally afflicted with gall-stones I should be more inclined to use "Dutch Drops," otherwise known as Oil of Haarlem,* in place of the olive oil; and this because I have known Dutch Drops to cure gall-stones after a variety of treatments had been previously and unsuccessfully tried. It is very probable, however, that Molasses would enhance the treatment. It is also probable that the inclusion of Molasses in one's daily diet would act as a preventive.

* Oil of Haarlem consists of sulphurated oil with a little refined turpentine.

14
NERVE CASES

The effects of the Molasses-treatment on bad nerves and war-neurosis have been so pronounced that the wives of soldiers returned from the war have noticed the striking improvement in their husbands and have expressed their gratitude for all that Molasses has done for these unfortunate sufferers. As for nervous children, they have benefited so greatly that whole families are now being given daily doses of the aliment as an adjunct to their diet. The treatment has not only benefited their nerves but has also made them healthier and stronger in every way.

15
PREGNANCY.
CHANGE OF LIFE

Many prospective mothers who have been advised to take Molasses during the term of pregnancy have not only had easy confinements but have given birth to unusually healthy infants.

The menopause is said to be, and often *is*, a very difficult time with women. But this, in a large number of cases, must be attributed to years of wrong feeding, and a deficiency of mineral salts and vitamins. It is, therefore not surprising to hear that the Molasses-treatment has proved of enormous value to women at this critical period of their lives.

16
UNHEALTHY FINGER NAILS. THE HAIR

Dr. Forbes Ross, in his book on Cancer, mentioned the beneficial effect of potassium salts on brittle and crumbling finger nails. Similar effects have been observed after taking Molasses for even a week or two; brittle or crumbling nails having regained their firmness. There is also, in many cases, a noticeable improvement in the hair; a fact which Dr. Forbes Ross likewise mentioned in connection with his potassium treatment.* Some women who had been prematurely grey, were even wrongly accused of resorting to hairdye, seeing that their hair had regained its original

* See Appendix 1, para. 2; also Appendix II.

colour. Indeed the fact that the taking of Molasses should in some instances restore the pigment of the hair opens up a new field for speculation and investigation as to the real cause of premature greyness—unless attributable to shock or intense grief. For it shows that grey hair must be primarily due to a lack of some particular ingredient in the human body, an ingredient which is present in Molasses. To assume, however, that the missing ingredient was potassium alone would not be safe, in that Molasses contains other salts; and so did the Forbes Ross formula for growths—it contained, among other things, a certain small percentage of iron, though he considered the potash the most important..... But I will not enlarge on this matter.

17
THE EFFECT OF MOLASSES AFTER OR BEFORE SURGICAL INTERFERENCE

A man with a large lump below the knee (diagnosed as cancer) decided to have it extirpated. But prior to the operation he was induced to take a course of the Molasses-treatment. The subsequent speedy and perfect healing of the wound was commented on by his physicians. This is no isolated case. Mr. Persson informs me that judging from many reliable reports received, the evidence goes to show that when surgery has been resorted to for one reason or another, the healing processes have been much facilitated and accelerated when the patient has taken a course of Molasses prior to and following the operation.

Here is another instructive case: A woman was operated on for the removal of a lump, presumably thought to be cancerous. Before the operation she had been taking Molasses for some time; with the result that the growth was "dead," and when the surgeon came to use the knife, it was only hanging on by a mere thread . . . . This case, if it really was malignant, is instructive in view of what Dr. Forbes Ross pointed out over thirty years ago, namely that by means of the potassium treatment, growths lost their malignancy and became, so to say, dead; in which case an operation, if necessary at all, was a much easier matter and far less likely to lead to a recurrence as the result of scarred tissue which provides a fertile soil for malignancy if the blood and cells are deficient in potassium salts. What we always need to remember in this connection is that surgery merely deals with an effect and not with the prime cause, and hence it is not surprising that under orthodox treatment there is sooner or later a return of the original disease in the form of a new growth.

Which brings us to the following reflections.

18
"PREVENTION IS BETTER THAN CURE"

The truth of this hackneyed old saying has been twisted and exploited for insidious commercial purposes on the disregarded assumption that one can "prevent" a thing which nobody can be certain is bound to occur. This would not matter much if the alleged preventives were entirely harmless. But unfortunately many of the vaccines and serums now used in orthodox medicine have in a number of cases either immediate or long-delayed after-effects of a harmful nature. The trouble is, however, that just as it is impossible to prove save by circumstantial evidence that so-termed prophylactics do not prevent what might never have happened in any case, so it is impossible to prove save by circumstantial evidence their long-delayed undesirable after-effects. For instance, I recently heard from a naturopath in Australia that since an increasing number of children in that continent have been immunized against diphtheria, there has been a considerable increase in cases of infantile paralysis among the child population. Now it is a significant fact that immunization in many isolated cases has been known to cause paralysis, sometimes lasting for a whole week in the newly immunized. This being the case, can it be ruled out that instead of paralysis occurring immediately, and eventually passing off, the action of the serum may be delayed and give rise at a later date to that more intractable form termed infantile paralysis?

It may now be asked what bearing has all this on Molasses and the old adage quoted above? Is it to be inferred that I am going so far as to maintain that Molasses will prevent smallpox, typhoid, diphtheria and all the other acute diseases which vaccines are said to prevent? Yet granted that acute diseases are much less likely to occur when the blood and tissues are kept in a healthy state through absorbing the requisite vitamins and mineral salts, the type of prevention with which we are here concerned is of quite a different order. To illustrate my point I will again refer to Dr. Forbes Ross, and at this juncture, to his noteworthy experience in connection with cancer. For during the whole of his years of practice he noticed that not one of his many regular patients ever developed malignancy; and he attributed this to the fact that he freely used potassium in his prescriptions, a policy which no other doctor, to his knowledge, had adopted. Here then we have, not the proof, but at any rate circumstantial evidence that potassium salts prevent cancer—though

(I for my part would add) provided that no other powerful causes are present.

The inference should be obvious. As Molasses is especially rich in potash and other valuable salts, it is reasonable to conclude from the circumstantial evidence that the habitual consumption of it would tend to prevent cancer, and such other diseases for which it has proved to be a cure. Moreover, as every naturopath knows, it is always best to absorb the required salts and vitamins from the foods we eat or the beverages we drink, rather than from medicaments, which, when all is said, are artificial products, extracts or what not, divorced from their natural environment. Wisely did the homoeopath, Dr. Dorothy Shepherd, who has written many enlightening books, give utterance to the dictum, "Let your foods be your medicines," and also, one might add, your prophylactics. Indeed the matter is of so much importance that I may quote from a letter recently received; though sad to relate it is only one out of many I have had in the same vein since writing my books on therapeutics. After informing me that the patient concerned was removed to hospital in order to be treated for cancer, my correspondent goes on to say:

"She died in the hospital after nine months' suffering, patiently borne. She had the usual hospital treatment—mainly 'dopes' to ease the pain. In this large hospital there was no special diet for cancer sufferers—indeed, all the patients seemingly are given the same food. Even a patient just operated on for appendicitis is given suet pudding if that is the 'sweet' of the day.

"This poor lady's fatal illness was my first experience of cancer, and I was amazed at the shortcomings of the present treatment of sufferers from that dire disease.

The lady in question had previously had a breast removed in the same hospital. No advice was given to help to prevent a recurrence of the disease, and within a year she was back in the hospital suffering from further cancerous growths, this time considered inoperable.

"Although the hospital doctors knew her case to be hopeless, a belt was ordered by them to ease pain in her spine. She was never able to wear it, and her husband (a working man) was charged fifteen guineas for it.

"A month before her death she was.... operated on.... In spite of her entreaties for an anaesthetic that would render her unconscious during the operation, only a local one was given 'because they had to study the muscle reflexes.' She complained of terrible pain during the operation, throughout which she was fully conscious, and was told that a second operation might be necessary within ten days, which filled her with despondency. After this first operation (when she was probably merely opened up to see the extent of the growth) her relatives were told that the hospital was most hopeful of her improvement under the new treatment. The second operation was not carried out."

There are thousands of such sad cases, and, alas, there will be thousands more until the orthodox Medical Profession begin to look further afield and to realize, as did Dr. Forbes Ross, that cancer, like many other diseases, is most frequently due to a lack and not the presence of some "unknown quantity" in the human organism, and that merely to operate or to burn the outward manifestation with radium is not to get rid of a cause but only to tinker with an effect. Admittedly, when the disease has made such inroads that death would ensue in a matter of a few weeks or less, then the knife becomes necessary in the hope that life may be prolonged. But unless the surgeon and his confreres possess some knowledge which enables them to advise the patient how to prevent a recurrence, the evil hour of even greater suffering is, in many cases, merely postponed, as in the sad example already mentioned. Is it not a noteworthy fact that many physicians who are not hidebound by orthodox, dogmatical views about cancer, have come to the conclusion, in company with naturopaths and biochemic practitioners, that growths are due to wrong feeding; by which they mean habitual consumption of refined and deficiency-foods, as Dr. Forbes Ross was one of the first to contend. White bread, white sugar and *boiled* vegetables are all deficiency foods; and yet for generations these have been the staple diet, plus cooked or tinned meat, of the majority of the population. As to the brownish bread which people are now obliged to eat, it is so little better than white bread, and perhaps in some respects worse, that it certainly does not make up for other deficiencies. It is true that a much better type of proper brown bread is procurable, but for some strange reason the man in the street dislikes the wholemeal loaf and won't be seen eating it. Consequently, as Drs. Bicknell and Prescott point out in their impressive book *The Vitamins in Medicine;* as the most valuable part of the grain is removed from flour and given to pigs and livestock, "the daily bread of the poor becomes a broken reed instead of the staff of life."

67

19
MOLASSES COULD
SOLVE THE PROBLEM

How, then is the problem to be solved? If people will not or can not live on a well-balanced diet, which, as every naturopath knows, is the secret of health provided there is no interference from disruptive emotions, then the best thing to do is to consume as a daily habit at least one food which contains the largest proportion of essentials to keep the blood and cells in a healthy condition, thus acting as a prophylaxis against the chronic disorders enumerated in these pages. From what has already been written it will have become obvious that the food in question is Crude Black Molasses. In addition to the valuable salts content, cane-sugar Molasses, contains 700 international units per hundred (approximately 3½ ounces) of Vitamin B2. As for the mineral salts, a rough analysis of one specimen used in this country for making silage, revealed 9 per cent. of these necessary substances. The precentage, however, is probably higher in the Molasses used in Australia and New Zealand for the same purpose and for the therapeutical purposes to which my correspondent, Mr. Persson, has drawn attention. This substance is almost as thick as putty and tastes much less sweet than the Molasses I have tasted here in England. In U.S.A. the Molasses used for making gingerbreads, etc., is termed blackstrap Molasses, and I note from a cutting in the "Daily Scotsman" (August 23rd, 1946) that the International Emergency Food Council announced that the 1946 allotment was 368,000,000 gallons, of which 103,200,000 gallons were allocated to the United Kingdom.

But now comes the snag. Despite this enormous allotment, Molasses is not at present available in this country for the general public but is reserved for the farmers. Whether it will have become available by the time this booklet is in print, I cannot pretend to predict, seeing that letters to the Board of Trade have evoked the reply that there is no medical evidence to hand that Molasses has ever been used in Great Britain for therapeutical purposes. And that may well be the case, for although some doctors may have heard of the valuable properties in Molasses, especially if they have read "The Vitamins in Medicine," that by no means proves they have advocated its consumption; orthodox physicians usually preferring to tell their patients what they should **not** eat rather than what they **should**. But in any case everything must have a beginning! After all there were times when certain herbs, foods and drugs we now know to contain valuable properties were looked upon as either useless or neutral—which is much the same thing. I can remember that, in the days of my boyhood, fruits were regarded by many people as nothing but luxuries, very often indigestible ones at that. Few doctors knew about the value of apples (which contain malic acid), and of the citric fruits which are now said to be useful against bacterial invasion. As for vitamins, about which we now hear so much, no such word existed and had not been even dreamt of by the scientist, though naturopaths did at least talk of "vital foods." And what about white sugar? It was thought to be that particular portion of the sugar-cane which was suitable for human consumption, whereas the Molasses, the other portion containing all the mineral salts of which doctors had never heard, was considered only fit to be given to livestock. The machinations of the sugar refiners last century may have been largely responsible for this, seeing they induced an unscrupulous doctor to "find" a "bug" in unrefined sugar which he conveniently alleged was harmful for human beings, though apparently it caused no trouble to animals! As matters now stand, the Molasses imported into this country for silage is labelled "Not Fit for Human Consumption," yet when a doctor who was interested in Molasses-therapy had a sample analysed, this analysis revealed nothing whatever of a harmful nature either to animal or to *man*. Whether the ruling on the part of the authorities is still based on the "bug" notion, I have been unable to ascertain. What is perhaps more likely is that as long as the imported aliment is labelled as above-mentioned, then less care has to be taken about the containers in which the substance is shipped.

20
WHITE SUGAR:
ACID-FORMING.
MOLASSES: ALKALINE.

I shall be doing no damage to the white sugar industry when I voice the dictum of food chemists that white sugar tends to create acidity; for just as people *will* eat white bread (when they can get it), so will they eat white sugar in preference to brown, however much they may be told that the latter is much more salubrious. Nor will they refrain from eating white sugar when they are told that it is conductive to rheumatism and distinctly bad for the teeth, as opposed to Molasses which tends to preserve the teeth, and, having a somewhat alkaline action, helps to ward off rheumatism and even to cure it. Furthermore, far from containing a harmful "bug," it has been shown to contain a germicide which destroys harmful bacteria in the intestinal tract. These facts having been put forward by food chemists and food specialists, the rational thing to do is to mix a little Molasses with all our jams and marmalade, just as an artist mixes his medium with his paints. In other words, white sugar having been deprived of its most essential and wholesome elements, these should be put back in the manner above indicated.

21
UNAVAILABLE IS NOT THE SAME AS UNOBTAINABLE

It will doubtless be argued: "What is the use of telling us all this when Molasses in this country is unavailable for the general public?" To which I repeat what has already been implied: (1) that this state of affairs may not continue when times become more normal and when sufficient public attention has been drawn to the curative value of Molasses; (2) that unavailable does not mean precisely the same thing as unobtainable. It is permissible, I understand, for any one person in Australia, New Zealand, Canada or other countries where procurable, to send a certain number of lbs. of the aliment per month to any given person in Great Britain.

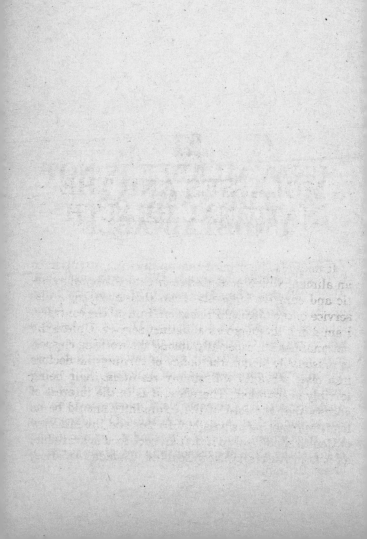

22
MOLASSES AND THE NATIONAL HEALTH

It may also be argued that in drawing attention to an aliment which possesses such extensive prophylactic and curative elements, I am thereby doing a disservice to the Medical Profession. But, on the contrary, I am doing its members a distinct service. Unless the national health, especially among the working classes, is reasonably sound, the policy of turning the doctors into civil servants will simply result in their being terribly overworked. Therefore, it is in the interest of doctors that the food of the community should be as health-promoting as possible. To this end the Ministry of Health should see to it that all such food is available, as it is in Australia, New Zealand, Canada, America, and other countries that could be mentioned. It is interesting to note that in Palmerston, N.Z., where Mr. Persson has for nine years been supplying large quantities of Molasses of the best and crudest kind, the latest statistics record a lower death rate and a greater population.

23
SUGAR-CANE: A LIFE-SUSTAINING FOOD IN ITSELF

The following information was given to me by a lady who has recently returned from India, where an associate of hers owned a cane-sugar plantation. She told me that some of the workers in the plantation were so poor, and that food was at times so scarce, that they were obliged to live on and to feed their children on sugar-cane exclusively. They ate all but the fibres, which they ejected; and on this mono-diet contrived to sustain life and remain healthy.

24
METHOD OF TAKING MOLASSES

The most convenient way of taking Molasses is before meals. The dosage is one teaspoonful, which should be melted in half a cup of hot water, then cold water should be added, so as to make two-thirds of a cupful, the latter to be drunk warm. For children, half the dosage. The Molasses *can* be taken neat; but hot water should be drunk immediately afterwards. Some people, however find the latter method unsuited to them. The patient must use his own judgment and adapt the method to his individual idiosyncracies. Persons with delicate stomachs who find a teaspoonful too much at one time, should take a smaller dose but more often during the day. In severe cases, such as for growths,

Molasses should be taken last thing at night and on rising, as well as during the day. The water should of course never be too hot; never hotter than a temperature in which one can comfortably bear to put one's finger. It is the utmost folly to drink any beverage scaldingly hot, like some persons drink tea. Another point is that the Molasses-and-water mixtures should not be gulped down like nasty medicine so as to produce flatulence, but should be sipped and tasted like connoisseurs taste good wines. The reason for taking the Molasses in hot water is because by being thus diluted it is more easily assimilated, and also more digestible. Cold water with some people is apt to chill the stomach. Even bladder troubles can occur after people have drunk draughts of cold water at a time when they are over-heated.

Both children and adults can, with advantage, take Molasses in the milk they use with their porridge or dry cereals for breakfast or at other times. I have already mentioned how a little Molasses may be and should be mixed with marmalade and all jams made from white sugar. I have also mentioned how Molasses should be taken per rectum in cases of growths in the bowels, or colitis, etc. For external growths, boils, sores, cuts, etc., Molasses mixed with water should be applied as a poultice, in addition to the internal treatment. As a natural ointment Molasses has no equal.

The reader is warned against the use of the *medicated* variety sold in tins in U.S.A. and elsewhere. People who have tried this stuff have complained of discomfort in the stomach. In any case it is unwise to take medicated aliments over a long period. In asking friends in U.S.A. to send Molasses, it is therefore important to state that other than *unsulphured blackstrap* Molasses should *not* be dispatched. I should add that people in this country (England) have rather vague notions as to what the name Molasses really denotes. Many individuals seem to think it is a synonym for Black Treacle. This, however, is incorrect, or at best misleading. The "Universal English Dictionary" defines the aliment as "the thick non-crystallizable dark syrup which drains from raw sugar during manufacture; thickest kind of treacle." Nevertheless, ordinary black treacle, such as Fowler's, is not Molasses, good though it is, for the reason that it is not the *thickest* kind; it is much richer in sugar than the type of Molasses most suited for therapeutical purposes. The very best type for this purpose is, as I mentioned before, almost as thick as putty; moreover it has a somewhat garlicky smell, and is rather more bitter than sweet, as well as tasting slightly salty. However, as the only sample of this variety I have so far tasted comes from New Zealand, and hence takes a long time to arrive, the blackstrap type will serve as the next best.

The above was written before I came to realise that there seems to be some confusion in U.S.A. about the nomenclature of Molasses. One correspondent writes me that Blackstrap Molasses is the trade name given to a particular brand, whereas another correspondent writes that it is a term for crude black molasses in general. Further to add to the confusion, an American friend tells me that in some States the molasses used by farmers is called sorgum. In the circumstances it is therefore difficult to give my American readers any accurate information.

CONCLUSION

It may be thought that I have made too many claims for this "wonder-food," so I will conclude with a note of warning. That great German naturopath, Louis Kuhne,* maintained that he could cure all diseases with his therapy but that he *could not cure all patients*. His meaning should become obvious as soon as we reflect that to say we cure a disease is only a half-truth, for what we really mean is that we cure an individual ... or should do, if we are not incompetent bunglers and he is curable at all. Now not only are no claims made that Molasses-therapy can cure every disease, but no claim is even made that it can cure all patients suffering from the disorders mentioned in these pages.

*Neo-Naturopathy The New Science of Healing by Louis Kuhne. Published by Benedict Lust Publications, P.O. Box 404, New York, N.Y. 10156.

If a patient resorts to Molasses-therapy when it is already too late, it stands to reason that he cannot be cured. Nevertheless, numerous patients have been restored to health by this natural and harmless means when orthodox methods have entirely failed. Many letters have been received from grateful erstwhile sufferers—among them doctors and clergymen—saying that "since taking Molasses I am an entirely new man." The reason is obvious to students of biochemistry and dietetics; such people having fed on deficiency foods have then taken Molasses and thereby, perhaps for the first time in their lives, have supplied the essential elements which their bodies needed. All the same, if they discontinue taking Molasses, they are likely in the course of time to suffer again, for potassium salts are the salts in particular which require constant replenishing; moreover, as biochemists point out, they are the most soluble salts (especially pot. phos.) and are easily lost when foods are cooked or boiled. Hence the advisability of taking Molasses at any rate once or twice a day even when in good health should be emphasized. This is all the more imperative, because, in addition to the deficiency-diet on which the majority of people live, the consumption of salty and soda-impregnated foods has vastly increased of late years. To this fact Dr. Henty Smalpage (Australia) attributes the much greater prevalence of tumours, cysts and cancerous growths. His contentions in his book on "Cancer," if considered in conjunction with those of the late Dr. Forbes Ross, are highly significant. If the sodium salts absorbed from soda-impregnated foods in far too large quantities, and also the table salt used as a condiment, are not counteracted by potassium salts constantly replenished there is the liability of growths or arthritis developing. The reason is that all this unusable amount of soda is not eliminated via the kidneys, but manifests as a "lump" in some people or as that debilitating condition termed rheumatoid arthritis. Potassium salts, however, effect this elimination and thus the danger is greatly minimized.

The most natural way of getting these salts into the system is by taking Crude Black Molasses.

NOTE:

Since writing the above, some significant case-histories have come to hand from Mr. Victor S. Welsford, of South Africa, who is doing much valuable service in the interest of health. Here is an arthritis case. Gentleman; in bed for three months with rheumatoid arthritis of such severity that he could hardly move his arms and hands. After having fifty electric and thermal treatments, he was informed that nothing more could be done for him. He then started Molasses therapy, with the result that after 3—4 months his health is in so far normal that he merely experiences slight twinges of pain in wet weather. Mr. Welsford further reports the case of a lady whose state was so serious that after resorting to Molasses, "she seems to be arising practically from a condition leading to death...."

APPENDIX

I
Extracts from the late Dr. Forbes Ross's book, "Cancer: Its Cause and Cure" long out of print.

(1) "The negroes of the West Indies on sugar plantations who have in the past shown a singular immunity from cancer, have always been most prodigious consumers of crude sugar. Crude sugar contains a large proportion of potassium salts, which for the most part is removed from the white or refined article. Being convinced from experience that the alkaline balance was really a matter of the amount of potassium present in the blood, I proceeded to work on the lines of taking care of the potassium supply of the body and leaving the sodium, calcium and magnesium to look after themselves, because whatever happened their supply at any time would be kept up by food and drink, so that it was

only necessary to attend to the supply of the one salt which was likely to vary in quantity to the other salts in the body, that salt being potassium."*

(2) "We will now consider the action of potassium on the hair. If an elderly person, suffering from gout, failure of the heart, or cancer, be made for a certain length of time, say six weeks, to artificially take into his or her body, a definite and ordered amount of potassium, the following change in the hair will certainly take place. If the hair be previously grey or iron grey it will become generally darker. The first localities of the scalp which will be found to show this change, in white or grey hair, will be a darkening of colour on the temples and the nape of the neck. These preliminary changes will be followed by the appearance of some normally coloured new hairs throughout the whole extent of the scalp, with the exception of those parts which had ceased to have any hair bulbs from which hair could possibly grow. So striking is the change that many elderly lady patients have been accused by their friends and relations of resorting to artifice to produce the resultant darkening and hair rejuvenescence as a result of taking potassium salts."

"The next point was that at first the scales which were removable from the skin of the body by friction with the hands or towel after the bath, were at first increased in quantity, and then occurred a gradual diminution of the total amount of epithelial scales lost from the surface of the skin, which then gradually sank to only that loss associated with younger persons."

"... The therapeutic agent that will cure cancer will be an agent which forms a natural constituent of the body in health, and therefore one which the body under conditions of disease will make use of to return to conditions of health. The body can only make use naturally of a natural means or force to effect the spontaneous cure of any disease. No medicinal treatment known to man is ever successful unless the body makes use of one of its natural means as the result of that medicinal treatment in order to return to healthy condition. No disease, whether spontaneously cured or by means of drugs, ever recovers except by reason of the natural forces and constituents of the body...."

II

As, according to analysis, Molasses contains pantothenic acid, some further reflections on this factor of the Vitamin B complex may prove instructive. Pantothenic acid (as the name implies) is widely distributed in both the vegetable and animal kingdoms. It has sometimes been called "yeast-growth substance," or "chick-antidermatitis factor"; and when there is a deficiency of it in the animal organism, skin, feathers, hair, as also the gastro-intestinal and respiratory systems are adversely affected. In rats the deficiency leads to the greying of the fur, and in mice to baldness. After using synthetic pantothenic acid, plus some other ingredients, on human subjects, certain American researchers noticed such effects as growth of new hair, a more healthy and lustrous appearance of the hair together with a tendency towards a reversion to its original colour. Thus it would seem that pantothenic acid acts to some extent as a "hair restorer." But if so, it is not exclusively the pantothenic acid, seeing that before this substance was discovered, grey hair in some cases reverted to its original colour as the result of taking potassium, in accordance with Dr. Forbes Ross's formula. And so where Molasses has likewise acted as a natural hair restorer, it is not unreasonable to assume that the effect has been produced by the combination of potassium and pantothenic acid, whilst probably the iron and copper in Crude Black Molasses have also been contributing factors.

It is interesting to note that, according to a brief report in the J.A.M.A. (November 24th, 1945), Dr. W. Stepp, of Munich, had been successfully employing synthetic pantothenic for chronic bronchitis. But, as the late Dr. Clarke, of Edinburgh, wrote some years ago vitamins, etc., should be absorbed from the foods we eat. Dame Nature is a better chemist than the scientist!

ANALYSIS OF SUGAR BEET MOLASSES (IRISH)

Water	... ... 21.9%
Albuminoids	... ... 10.5%
Carbohydrates	... ... 60.4%
Ash	... ... 7.2%

100% Starch Eq. 48.

Rich in Potassium. Poor in Calcium and Phosphorous.

With all due respect to Dr. Forbes Ross, it is doubtful whether the majority of people do absorb a sufficiency of calcium and magnesium salts from the foods they eat, hence they would be well advised to include Molasses in their daily diet, seeing it is not only rich in potassium salts but also in calcium, magnesium and iron; in a word, it is the "perfect food."

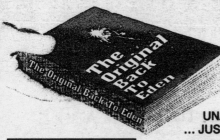